American College of Surgeons
Protocol for Cancer Surgery Documentation: Adrenal Cancer

Name: ACS.CSSP.protocol.adernal.2024.v1

What This Protocol Includes and Covers

- A synoptic operative report for adrenal cancer surgery
  - Section 1: EMR Autopopulated Information
  - Section 2: Cancer-Specific Information *(required)*
  - Section 3: Additional Procedure Details
- The synoptic operative report summary template
- Knowledge Platform with explanatory notes

American College of Surgeons Standards References

The following ACS standards references are heavily leveraged throughout the synoptic operative report and Knowledge Platform: *AJCC Cancer Staging Manual,* Eighth Edition; *Operative Standards for Cancer Surgery,* Volume 3; and *Standards for Oncology Registry Entry (STORE) 2023*.

Authors

Barbra S. Miller, MD, FACS*; Marybeth S. Hughes, MD, FACS*; Amanda M. Laird, MD, FACS*; Matthew A. Nehs, MD, FACS*

Reviewers

Paxton V. Dickson, MD, FACS†; Benzon Dy, MD, FACS†; Colleen M. Kiernan, MD, MPH, FACS†; Alexander Kutikov, MD, FACS†; Nancy D. Perrier, MD, FACS†; Heather Wachtel, MD, FACS†

Contributors

Herbert Chen, MD, FACS; Michael J. Demeure, MD, MBA, FACS, FACE; Gerard M. Doherty, MD, FACS; Quan-Yang Duh, MD, FACS; Douglas B. Evans, MD, FACS; Douglas L. Fraker, MD, FACS; Thomas J. Giordano, MD, PhD; Raymon H. Grogan, MD, MS, FACS; Elizabeth G. Grubbs, MD, FACS; Gary D. Hammer, MD, PhD; Marybeth S. Hughes, MD, FACS; Electron Kebebew, MD, FACS; Jennifer H. Kuo, MD, MS, FACS; Jeffrey E. Lee, MD, FACS; Travis McKenzie, MD, FACS; Sarah C. Oltmann, MD, FACS; Jennifer E. Rosen, MD, FACS; Allan Siperstein, MD; Carmen C. Solorzano, MD, FACS, FSSO; Tracy S. Wang, MD, MPH, FACS

**Denotes primary author. †Denotes synoptic operative report reviewer.*

Synoptic Operative Report

What This Synoptic Operative Report Covers and Includes
This synoptic operative report (SOR) covers documentation for adrenal cancer surgery.

The SOR includes roughly 15 fields for EMR autopopulated data, 19 fields for tumor-specific data (required), and 3 fields for additional procedure data that assist with billing and regulatory and practice requirements. This SOR was designed for cases of primary adrenal malignancy and not for benign disease. However, narrative text boxes may facilitate expanded use of this synoptic report at the user's discretion.

How This Synoptic Operative Report Is Organized
Required fields are indicated by an asterisk (*).

Section 1: EMR Autopopulated Information

Patient Name*
Patient ID*
Date of Surgery*
Name of Surgeon*
Name of Co-Surgeon
Name of Assistant(s)
Indication for Surgery*
Preoperative Diagnosis*
Postoperative Diagnosis*
Procedure(s) Performed*
Specimens Removed
Type of Anesthesia
Estimated Blood Loss
Drain/Implant
Additional Administrative Details

Section 2: Tumor-Specific Information *(required)*

Biochemical Testing Preformed*
Distant Metastatic Disease by Preoperative Imaging*
Evidence of Clinical Adenopathy*
Suspected Extra-Adrenal Extension of Tumor into Periadrenal Fat*
Suspected Extension to Adjacent Organs*
Suspected Vascular Invasion of Vessel Wall (with or without Thrombus)*
Venous Tumor Thrombus*
Procedure(s) Performed*
Approach*
Complete Exploration of Peritoneal Cavity*
Inclusion of Periadrenal Adipose Tissue with Specimen*
Adjacent Organs Resected if Invasion Suspected*
Lymph Nodes Removed*
Venous Thrombectomy*
Venous Reconstruction*
Need for Vascular Bypass*
Resection of Metastatic Disease*
Capsular Disruption of Tumor*
Clinical Resection Status*

Section 3: Additional Procedure Details

Additional Procedures
Additional Surgical Variables
Intraoperative Complications

Instructions

This report is intended for documentation at the completion of each surgical procedure.

Instructions are provided for each data field.

Explanatory notes provide reference material for each data field.

Narrative boxes are available in all sections of the SOR to allow the addition of provider-specific information as needed.

Completing all applicable data fields in the SOR will generate a SOR summary that is compliant with multiple regulatory requirements.

- **Section 1 Instructions:** You are being asked to review all the data fields in Section 1 as the information is autopopulated from the EMR and should be checked for accuracy. Please make corrections as needed and be sure to complete required fields. Throughout the tool, required fields are marked with an asterisk (*) and represent best practice.
- **Section 2 Instructions:** You are asked to complete all data fields in this section (Tumor-Specific Information) because they are required as part of best practice.
- **Section 3 Instructions:** You are not required to complete these data fields, but the additional surgical data elements included in this section (Additional Procedure Details) will support diverse coding, regulatory, and practice needs.

Section 1: EMR Autopopulated Information (Note A)

The following fields are standardized across all CSSPSORs.

Patient Name*
Patient ID*
Date of Surgery*
Name of Surgeon*
Name of Co-Surgeon
Name of Assistant(s)
Indication for Surgery*
Preoperative Diagnosis*
Postoperative Diagnosis*
Procedure(s) Performed*
Specimens Removed
Type of Anesthesia
Estimated Blood Loss
Drain/Implant
Additional Administrative Details

Section 2: Cancer-Specific Information (Note B)

Preoperative Assessment

*** Biochemical Testing Performed** (Note C)
Evidence of inappropriate hormone secretion (excess or mild autonomous secretion).
Select single best answer.
__ Yes
    [If yes is selected, display the following:]
    Select all that apply:
    __Cortisol
        __ Abnormal
        __ Normal
    __ACTH
        __ Abnormal
        __Normal
    __11-deoxycorticosteroids
        __Abnormal
        __Normal
    __Aldosterone
        __Abnormal
        __Normal
    __Androgens
        __Abnormal
        __Normal
    __DHEA-S
        __Abnormal
        __Normal
    __Androstenedione
        __Abnormal
        __Normal
    __Estrogens
        __Abnormal
        __Normal
    __17-OH Progesterone
        __Abnormal
        __Normal
    __Other – Describe *[Narrative Box]*
__ No

*** Distant Metastatic Disease by Preoperative Imaging** (Note D)
Select single best answer.
__ Yes
[If yes is selected, display the following:]
Select all that apply:
__Liver
__Lung
__Omentum
__Peritoneum
__Spleen
__Bone
__Extra-regional lymph nodes
__Soft tissue
__Brain
__Other – Describe *[Narrative Box]*
__ No

*** Preoperative Therapy** (Note E)
Select all that apply.
__ None
__ Systemic therapy
[If yes is selected, display the following:]
__ Chemotherapy
__ Immunotherapy
__ Other – Describe *[Narrative Box]*
__ Radiation therapy
__ Hormone targeted therapy (to lower/negate cortisol, aldosterone, sex hormone excess)
__ Preoperative antihypertensive medication (specifically to treat hormone or catecholamine excess)
__ Other – Describe *[Narrative Box]*

Intraoperative Findings

*** Evidence of Clinical Adenopathy** (Note F)
Select single best answer.
__ Yes
[If yes is selected, display the following:]
Location: Select all that apply.
__ Renal
__ Paracaval
__ Suprarenal
__ Infrarenal
__ Para-aortic
__ Suprarenal
__ Infrarenal
__ Interaortocaval
__ Celiac
__ Superior mesenteric vessels
__ Other – Describe [*Narrative Box*]

__ No

*** Suspected Extra-Adrenal Extension of Tumor into Periadrenal Adipose Tissue** (Note G)
Select single best answer.
__ Yes
__ No

*** Suspected Extension to Adjacent Organs** (Note H)
Select single best answer.
__ Yes
  [If yes is selected, display the following:]
  Select all that apply.
  __Colon
  __Stomach
  __Pancreas
  __Spleen
  __Liver
  __Diaphragm
  __Small Bowel
  __Duodenum
  __Gallbladder
  __Abdominal wall
  __ Peritoneal surface
  __Other –Describe *[Narrative Box]*
__ No

*** Suspected Vascular Invasion of Vessel Wall (with or without Thrombus** (Note I)
Select single best answer.

__ Yes
  [If yes is selected, display the following:]
  Select all that apply.
  __Renal vein
  __Renal artery
  __IVC
  __Celiac axis
  __ Aorta
  __Splenic artery
  __Hepatic artery
  __Portal vein
  __Superior mesenteric artery
  __Other –Describe *[Narrative Box]*
__ No

*** Venous Tumor Thrombusy** (Note J)
Select single best answer.
__ Yes
[If yes is selected, display the following:]
Location of thrombus
Select all that apply.
__ IVC
__ Right renal vein
__ Left renal vein
__Adrenal vein
__ Other – Describe [*Narrative Box*]

Distal extent of thrombus
Select all that apply:
__ Adrenal vein
__ Renal vein
__ Infrahepatic IVC
__ Retrohepatic IVC caudal to or at hepatic veins
__ Retrohepatic IVC cranial to hepatic veins
__ Suprahepatic at or below diaphragm
__ Suprahepatic above diaphragm
__ Intracardiac
__ Other—Describe extent (levels 1–4) [*Narrative Box*]
__ No

Operative Details

*** Procedure(s) Performed** (Note K)
Was the operation performed for curative intent? Select single best answer.
__ Yes
__ No
[If no is selected, display the following:]
Select single best answer.
__ Diagnostic intent [*Narrative Box*]
__ Palliative intent [*Narrative Box*]

Adrenal removed:
__Right adrenalectomy
__Left adrenalectomy
__Bilateral adrenalectomy

*** Approach** (Note L)
Select all that apply.
__ Open
__ Laparoscopic
[If "Laparoscopic" is selected, display the following:]
__ With hand assist
__ Without hand assist
__ Laparoscopic converted to open—Describe reason [*Narrative Box*]
__ Robot-assisted
__ Robot-assisted converted to open—Describe reason [*Narrative Box*]
__ Retroperitoneoscopic

*** Complete Exploration of Peritoneal Cavity** (Note M)
Select single best answer.
__ Yes
__ No

*** Inclusion of Periadrenal Adipose Tissue with Specimen** (Note N)
Select single best answer.
__ Yes
__ No

*** Adjacent Organs Resected if Suspected of Invasion** (Note O)
Select single best answer.
__ No
__ Yes
  [If yes is selected, display the following:]
  Organ(s) removed
  Select all that apply.
  __Kidney (Partial vs. total nephrectomy for invasion)
  __Colon
  __Stomach
    [If "Stomach" is selected, display the following:]
    __ Total
    __ Partial
  __Pancreas
  __Spleen
  __Liver
  __Diaphragm
  __Small Bowel
  __Duodenum
  __Gallbladder
  __Other – Describe [Narrative Box]
  En-bloc resection of above organs
  __ Yes
  __ No

*** Lymph Nodes Removed** (Note P)
Select single best answer.
__ Yes
  [If yes is selected, display the following:]
  __ Formal dissection
  __ Sampling
    [If "sampling" is selected, display the following:]
    Location(s) of nodes removed
    Select all that apply
    __ Renal
    __ Paracaval
      [If "Paracaval" is selected, display the following:]
      __ Suprarenal
      __ Infrarenal

__ Para-aortic
[If "Para-aortic" is selected, display the following:]
__ Suprarenal
__ Infrarenal
__ Interaortocaval
__ Celiac
__ Superior mesenteric artery
__ Other—Describe [*Narrative Box*]
__ No

*** Venous Thrombectomy** (Note Q)
Select single best answer.
__ Yes
__ No

*** Venous Reconstruction** (Note R)
Select single best answer.
__ Yes
[If yes is selected, display the following:]
__ Primary repair
__ Patch
__ Graft [*Narrative Box*]
__ No
[If no is selected, display the following:]
__Ligation of IVC

*** Need for Vascular Bypass** (Note S)
Select single best answer.
__ Yes
[If yes is selected, display the following:]
__ Venovenous
__ Cardio-pulmonary bypass with or without hypothermic circulatory arrest
__ No

*** Resection of Metastatic Disease** (Note T)
__ Yes –Describe location [*Narrative Box*]
[If yes is selected, display the following:]
Organs removed
Select all that apply.
__Kidney
[If "Kidney" is selected, display the following:]
__ Total (The entire kidney is removed.)
__ Partial (A portion of renal parenchyma is removed. This does not include removing the capsule of the kidney alone.)
__Colon
__Stomach
[If "Stomach" is selected, display the following:]
__ Total
__ Partial

__Pancreas
__Spleen
__Liver
[If "Liver" is selected, display the following:]
__ Formal anatomic resection (lobectomy, segmentectomy) is performed.
__ Partial (Non-anatomic resection is performed.)
__ Ablative or other destruction (Radiofrequency ablation, microwave ablation, cryoablation, other)
__Diaphragm
__Small Bowel
__Duodenum
__Gallbladder
__Peritoneal Lining
__Other – Describe [*Narrative Box*]
__ No

*** Capsular Disruption of Tumor** (Note U)
__ Yes
[If yes is selected, display the following:]
Gross Tumor spillage
__ Yes
__ No
__ No

*** Clinical Resection Status** (Note V)
Select single best answer.
__ R0/R1 (All evidence of tumor removed without visible or palpable evidence of residual in-situ tumor remaining at conclusion of case.)
__ R2 (Known visible or palpable tumor [whether by inspection or radiographic evidence] remains at conclusion of case.)

Section 3: Additional Procedure Details

Additional Procedures (Note W)
__ None
__ Yes—Describe [*Narrative Box*]

Additional Surgical Variables (Note X)
__ None
__ Yes—Describe [*Narrative Box*]
__ Provided elsewhere [*Narrative Box*]

Intraoperative Complications (Note Y)
__ None
__ Yes—Describe [*Narrative Box*]

SOR Summary Template (Mockup)

Adrenal Cancer

Patient Name: *[Autopopulate from EMR]*
Patient ID: *[Autopopulate from EMR]*
Date of Surgery: *[Autopopulate from EMR]*
Name of Surgeon: *[Autopopulate from EMR]*
Name of Co-Surgeon: *[Autopopulate from EMR]*
Name of Assistant(s): *[Autopopulate from EMR – Nurses notes]*
Indication for Surgery: *[Autopopulate from EMR; **or** override with EMR pick list]*
Preoperative Diagnosis: *[Autopopulate from EMR; **or** override with SOR selections]*
Postoperative Diagnosis: *[Autopopulate from EMR; **or** override with SOR selections]*
Procedure(s) Performed: *[Autopopulate from EMR; **or** override with SOR selections]*
Specimens Removed: *[Autopopulate from EMR – Nurses notes with override capability]*
Type of Anesthesia: *[Autopopulate from EMR – Anesthesia with override capability]*
Estimated Blood Loss: *[Autopopulate from EMR – Anesthesia with override capability]*
Drain/Implant *[Autopopulate from EMR – Nurses notes with override capability]*
Additional Administrative Details: *[Autopopulate from EMR; **or** Narrative text]*

Tumor-Specific Information
Preoperative Assessment
[Fill from SOR: <u>Biochemical Testing Performed</u>]
[Fill from SOR: <u>Distant Metastatic Disease by Preoperative Imaging</u>]
[Fill from SOR: <u>Preoperative Therapy</u>]
Intraoperative Findings
[Fill from SOR: <u>Evidence of Clinical Adenopathy</u> and if applicable <u>Location</u>]
[Fill from SOR: <u>Suspected Extra-Adrenal Extension of Tumor into Periadrenal Adipose Tissue</u>]
[Fill from SOR: <u>Suspected Extension to Adjacent Organs</u>]
[Fill from SOR: <u>Suspected Vascular Invasion of Vessel Wall (with or without Thrombus)</u>]
[Fill from SOR: <u>Venous Tumor Thrombus</u> and, if applicable, <u>Location of Thrombus</u> and <u>Distal Extent of Thrombus</u>]

Operative Details
[Fill from SOR: <u>Procedure(s) Performed</u>]
[Fill from SOR: <u>Approach</u>]
[Fill from SOR: <u>Complete Exploration of Peritoneal Cavity</u>]
[Fill from SOR: <u>Inclusion of Periadrenal Adipose Tissue with Specimen</u>]
[Fill from SOR: <u>Adjacent Organs Resected if Suspected of Invasion</u>]
[Fill from SOR: <u>Lymph Nodes Removed</u> and, if applicable, <u>Location(s) of Nodes Removed</u>]
[Fill from SOR: <u>Venous Thrombectomy</u>]
[Fill from SOR: <u>Venous Reconstruction</u>]
[Fill from SOR: <u>Need for Vascular Bypass</u>]
[Fill from SOR: <u>Resection of Metastatic Disease</u>]
[Fill from SOR: <u>Capsular Disruption of Tumor</u>]
[Fill from SOR: <u>Clinical Resection Status</u>]

Additional Procedure Details
[Fill from SOR: <u>Additional Procedures</u>]
[Fill from SOR: <u>Additional Surgical Variables</u>]
[Fill from SOR: <u>Intraoperative Complications</u>]

Knowledge Platform

Introductory Comments
This protocol is intended to standardize documentation and communication of critical components of adrenal cancer surgery. The following explanatory notes reference critical elements for cancer surgery as described in the *Operative Standards for Cancer Surgery,* Volume 3, and expert panel consensus.

Instructions

Each Explanatory Note is linked from a corresponding data element in the synoptic report above and contains additional materials and references that can be used to facilitate accurate completion of the report.

Section 1: EMR Autopopulated Information

Note A: EMR Autopopulated Information

Explanatory Comments: The following fields are intended to be prepopulated with site-specific identifiers and information from the EMR.

Patient Name
Patient ID
Date of Surgery
Name of Surgeon
Name of Co-Surgeon
Name of Assistant(s)
Indication for Surgery
Preoperative Diagnosis
Postoperative Diagnosis
Procedure(s) Performed
Specimens Removed
Type of Anesthesia
Estimated Blood Loss
Drain/Implant
Additional Administrative Details

Section 2: Cancer-Specific Information

Note B: Cancer-Specific Information

Explanatory Comments: This section of the SOR contains critical oncology data elements supported by evidence and best practice, as well as data fields defined by the *STORE* manual and submitted to hospital registries for NCDB and state registry reporting. There are data fields in this section related to findings and/or treatments in both the preoperative and intraoperative phases of care. To complete the preoperative data fields assumes that the patient has undergone comprehensive assessment which may include/includes physical examination, radiologic assessment, and adrenal specific biochemical testing.

Note C: Biochemical Testing Performed

Explanatory Comments: Preoperative evaluation of adrenal masses requires adrenal specific biochemical evaluation. This evaluation is to be consistent and comprehensive, and expanded to include various intermediaries along the steroid synthesis pathway. Indicate by selecting from the list which hormone levels were checked preoperatively. Selection of "abnormal" cortisol should be based on the final assessment of any autonomous cortisol production based on results of Dexamethasone suppression test (1mg dexamethasone suppression test with an a.m. cortisol of ≥ 1.8 mcg/dl (50 nmol/l) drawn between 0700 and 0800 with supporting evidence of a suppressed ACTH and an adequate quantitative dexamethasone level at the same time). Abnormal cortisol may also be indicated by an abnormal late night salivary cortisol or 24-hour urine cortisol above the upper limit of the institution's reference range. Aldosterone should be considered in the context of an accompanying renin level and confirmatory testing (if indicated) as primary aldosteronism may be diagnosed in the setting of aldosterone levels which fall within a laboratory's established normal range. If other adrenal-specific hormone testing was completed, please select "Other" and list the name of the hormone and if the result was normal or abnormal.

Note D: Distant Metastatic Disease by Preoperative Imaging

Explanatory Comments: Preoperative imaging may reveal evidence of distant metastatic disease. Please indicate any sites of distant metastatic disease according to the sites listed. If a focus on imaging is identified which remains indeterminate or too small to characterize and will be followed over time, please indicate this site under "Other" and note the finding is "indeterminate."

Note E: Preoperative Therapy

Explanatory Comments: In some patients with primary adrenal malignancies, systemic therapy may be administered as neoadjuvant therapy and other treatments or medications may be prescribed to control adrenal hormone excess. If the patient has received any of these treatments, select the appropriate item from the list provided. Medications to control adrenal hormone excess are included in Table 1.

Table 1. Medications to control adrenal hormone excess.

Hormone Excess	Medication
Cortisol	Metyrapone, Ketoconazole, Mifepristone, Etomidate, Mitotane, Osilodrostat
Aldosterone	Spironolactone, Eplerenone, Amiloride
Androgens	Spironolactone
Estrogens	Anastrozole

Note F: Evidence of Clinical Adenopathy

Explanatory Comments: This field documents data from clinical exams and/or imaging findings suggesting the presence of nodal metastases present before surgery. The type of imaging is not specified and could be any appropriate study. Nodal disease is defined as any lymph node noted on imaging review as indeterminate or concerning, has increased 18FDG avidity above the background, or is biopsy proven to be positive for metastatic disease. If imaging was performed and there was no evidence of nodal disease, the patient would be considered cN0. If there is evidence of nodal disease in any of the listed sites, the patient would be considered cN1. Physical exam does not suffice to define the patient as cN0 but could qualify the patient as cN1.

Note G: Suspected Extra-Adrenal Extension of Tumor into Periadrenal Adipose Tissue

Explanatory Comments: According to the AJCC staging system, extra-adrenal extension refers to the involvement of periadrenal adipose tissue, other soft tissue, adjacent organs, or direct extension of the tumor into the wall of adjacent vasculature (arterial or venous). Invasion beyond the adrenal tumor capsule that can be identified by imaging or intraoperative findings ranges from T3 disease (extension into periadrenal adipose tissue) to T4 disease (demonstrating gross extra-adrenal extension invading into nearby tissues or organs or venous tumor thrombus within the lumen of the vena cava or renal veins). If there is evidence supportive of the above-described extra-adrenal extension on any imaging studies performed (ultrasound, CT, MRI, PET imaging), select "yes." If the findings are negative for extra-adrenal extension, select "no." For additional details, please refer to the *Operative Standards for Cancer Surgery*, Volume 3, pages 73-142, and the *AJCC Cancer Staging Manual,* Eighth Edition.

Note H: Suspected Extension to Adjacent Organs

Explanatory Comments: At the time of operation, if there is suspected invasion or adherence to any of the listed organs or surfaces (peritoneum), please select the appropriate choice. According to the *AJCC Cancer Staging Manual,* Eighth Edition, extra-adrenal extension refers to the involvement of periadrenal adipose tissue, other soft tissue, adjacent organs, or direct extension of the tumor into the wall of adjacent vasculature (arterial or venous). Invasion beyond the adrenal tumor capsule that can be identified by imaging and is beyond extension into the periadrenal adipose tissue is denoted as T4 disease (demonstrating gross extra-adrenal extension invading into nearby tissues or organs or venous tumor thrombus within the lumen of the vena cava or renal veins). If evidence supports the above-described extra-adrenal extension on any imaging studies performed (ultrasound, CT, MRI, PET imaging), select "yes." If the findings are negative for extra-adrenal extension, select "no." If "indeterminate" on preoperative imaging, select "Other," list the site, and note as indeterminate invasion. For additional details, please refer to the *Operative Standards for Cancer Surgery,* Volume 3, pages 73-142, and the *AJCC Cancer Staging Manual,* Eighth Edition.

Note I: Suspected Vascular Invasion of Vessel Wall (with or without Thrombus)

Explanatory Comments: During resection, please indicate any artery or vein found to have evidence of direct invasion on imaging or that is involved by tumor thrombus. If the vessel is not listed, please use the narrative box to list any other named vasculature structures involved by tumor. According to the AJCC staging system, extra-adrenal extension involving adjacent vasculature is denoted as T4 disease. If there is evidence supportive of the above-described extra-adrenal extension on any preoperative imaging studies (ultrasound, CT, MRI, PET imaging), select "yes." If the findings are negative for extra-adrenal extension, select "no." If "indeterminate" on preoperative imaging, select "Other," list the site, and note as indeterminate invasion. For additional details, please refer to the *Operative Standards for Cancer Surgery,* Volume 3, pages 73-142, and the *AJCC Cancer Staging Manual,* Eighth Edition.

Note J: Venous Tumor Thrombus

Explanatory Comments: Venous tumor thrombus levels are stratified according to Figure 1. The distal extent refers to the most superior extent of venous tumor thrombus. Please indicate the level of distal extension of any venous tumor thrombus involving the renal veins or vena cava.

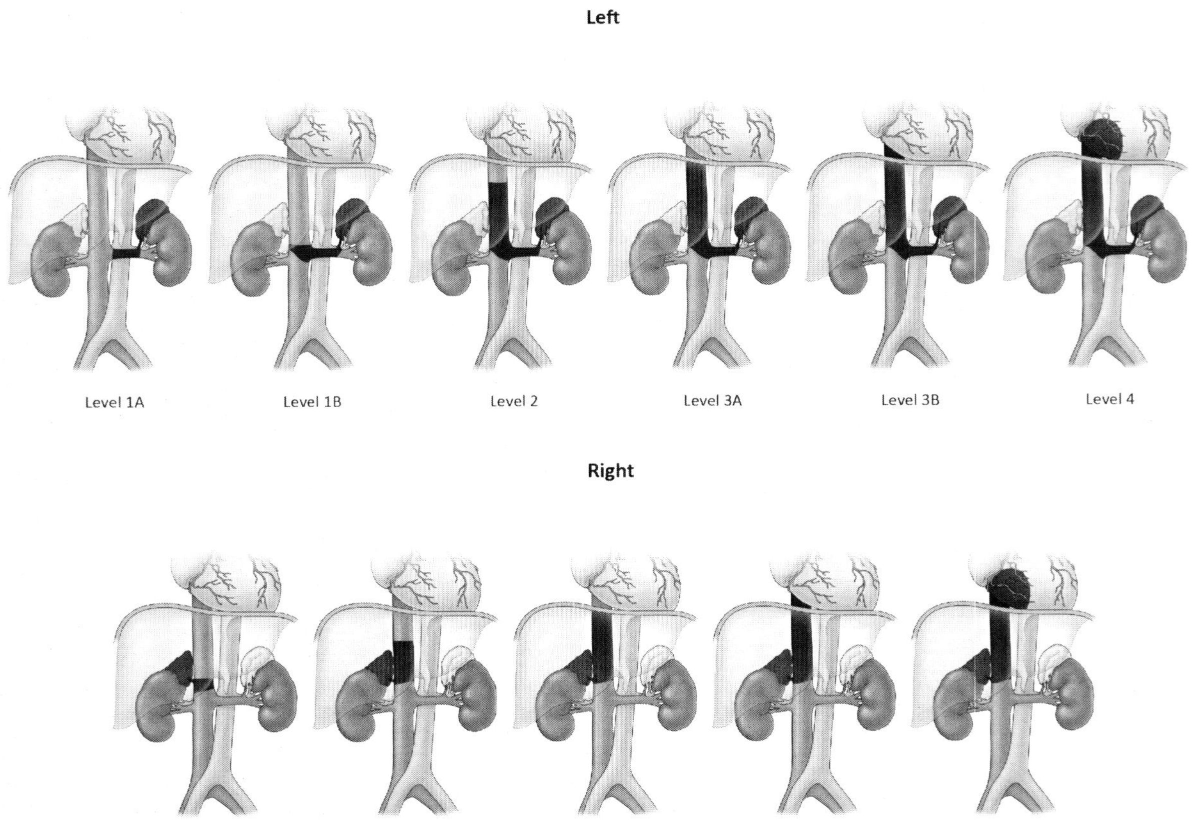

Figure 1 Venous Tumor Thrombus Extent. Left: Right: Level 1—extension of thrombus into the vena cava remaining at the level of the right adrenal vein or inferior to it; Level 2—extension of thrombus 2 cm or more superior to the adrenal vein yet still inferior to the hepatic veins; Level 3A—thrombus superior to the hepatic veins yet inferior to the diaphragm; Level 3B—thrombus extending superior to the diaphragm and no intracardicac involement; Level 4—thrombus within the atrium or beyond. Left: Level 1A-thrombus in the adrenal and/or renal vein only; Level 1B—thrombus exending into the vena cava not more than 2 cm superior to the renal vein-vena cava junction; Level 2—thrombus extending >2 cm into the infrahepatic vena cava and remaining inferior to the hepatic veins; Level 3A—thrombus extending superior to the hepatic veins and remaining inferior to the diaphragm; Level 3B—thrombus extending superior to the diaphragm and no intracardiac involvement; Level 4—thrombus within the atrium or beyond.

Note K: Procedure(s) Performed

Explanatory Comments: Indications for surgery and the intent of the planned surgery can be varied. Intent refers to surgery performed with the intent to cure the patient of their disease (resection to the point of no evidence of disease) versus intent to palliate the patient, leaving the patient with known residual disease. Select the intent of surgical resection. If surgery is to cure the patient of adrenal cancer, select "yes." If "no" is selected, please elaborate by selecting the next best choice. If there is not a diagnosis and the operation is carried out to determine histology, please mark as diagnostic intent. If known metastatic disease and operation is for cytoreduction or reduction of functional tumor burden, list as palliative intent. The adrenal gland, C74.0, and C74.9, currently falls under the surgical codes for "All Other Sites" as outlined in *STORE 2023*. This SOR only applies to adrenocortical cancers, not cancers originating from the medulla.

Note L: Approach

Explanatory Comments: Please indicate the most accurate description of the surgical approach. If an operation is started using a minimally invasive approach and converted to an open approach (beyond laparoscopic hand-assisted), please add reasons for conversion to an open approach in the narrative box.

This data field can be used to document the surgical approach used for the operation, which may be needed for certain billing and coding requirements.

NCDB codes are provided below in Table 2 for the Approach – Surgery of the Primary Site at this Facility (RxHospSurgApp 2010) [668] data item from *STORE 2023*.

Table 2. NCDB Codes for Approach – Surgery of the Primary Site at this Facility from *STORE* manual

NCDB Code	Label
0	No surgical procedure of primary site at this facility; Diagnosed at autopsy
1	Robot assisted
2	Robotic converted to open
3	Minimally invasive (such as retroperitoneoscopic or laparoscopic)
4	Minimally invasive (retroperitoneoscopic or laparoscopic) converted to open
5	Open or approach unspecified

ACS *STORE 2023* . Approach – Surgery of the Primary Site at this Facility (RxHospSurgApp 2010).

*This table has been amended to remove code 9 (unknown whether the surgery was performed at this facility) as it would not be an appropriate code in the context of this report.

Note M: Complete Exploration of Peritoneal Cavity

Explanatory Comments: As part of any abdominal operation for cancer, the peritoneal cavity should be thoroughly examined in a systematic manner, including bilateral upper and lower quadrants, and pelvis. Evidence of metastatic disease should be sought not only in the area of the primary tumor, but throughout the peritoneal cavity. Other abnormalities unrelated to the primary tumor should also be sought. At the time of surgical exploration, the visceral and parietal peritoneum should be evaluated for surface metastatic disease. The solid organs are palpated to assess for masses within, and if concern is noted, ultrasound may be utilized to interrogate further. If the entire peritoneal cavity has been explored, select "yes," and if no exploration or an incomplete exploration of the peritoneal cavity is performed, select "no." For additional details, please refer to the *Operative Standards for Cancer Surgery,* Volume 3, pages 73-142, and the *AJCC Cancer Staging Manual,* Eighth Edition.

Note N: Inclusion of Periadrenal Adipose Tissue with Specimen

Explanatory Comments: Given frequent capsular invasion by the tumor into surrounding periadrenal soft tissue, inclusion of periadrenal adipose tissue is a key technical step in the resection of adrenal cancer (OSCS). This facilitates negative margins and adequate tumor staging. T2 tumors are those confined by the tumor capsule, while according to the *AJCC Cancer Staging Manual*, Eighth Edition, tumor extension into the periadrenal adipose tissue defines T3 tumors. This leads to a change in stage from Stage 2 to Stage 3 resulting in potential changes in recommendations for adjuvant therapy. Inclusion of periadrenal adipose tissue is defined by resection of the retroperitoneal adipose tissue inferiorly from the level of the renal vein or sufficiently inferior to the adrenal gland to include periadrenal adipose tissue, laterally to the abdominal side wall, superiorly to the diaphragm, and medially over the anterior surface of the vena cava and soft tissue posterior to the vena cava. Marking sutures for orientation should mark this periadrenal soft tissue furthest from the tumor to indicate margins of resection to the pathologist. If periadrenal adipose tissue is included *en bloc* with the tumor, mark "yes." Mark "no" if the dissection described above has not been performed. For additional details, please refer to the *Operative Standards for Cancer Surgery,* Volume 3, pages 73-142, and the *AJCC Cancer Staging Manual,* Eighth Edition, Figure 2-2, pages 86-87.

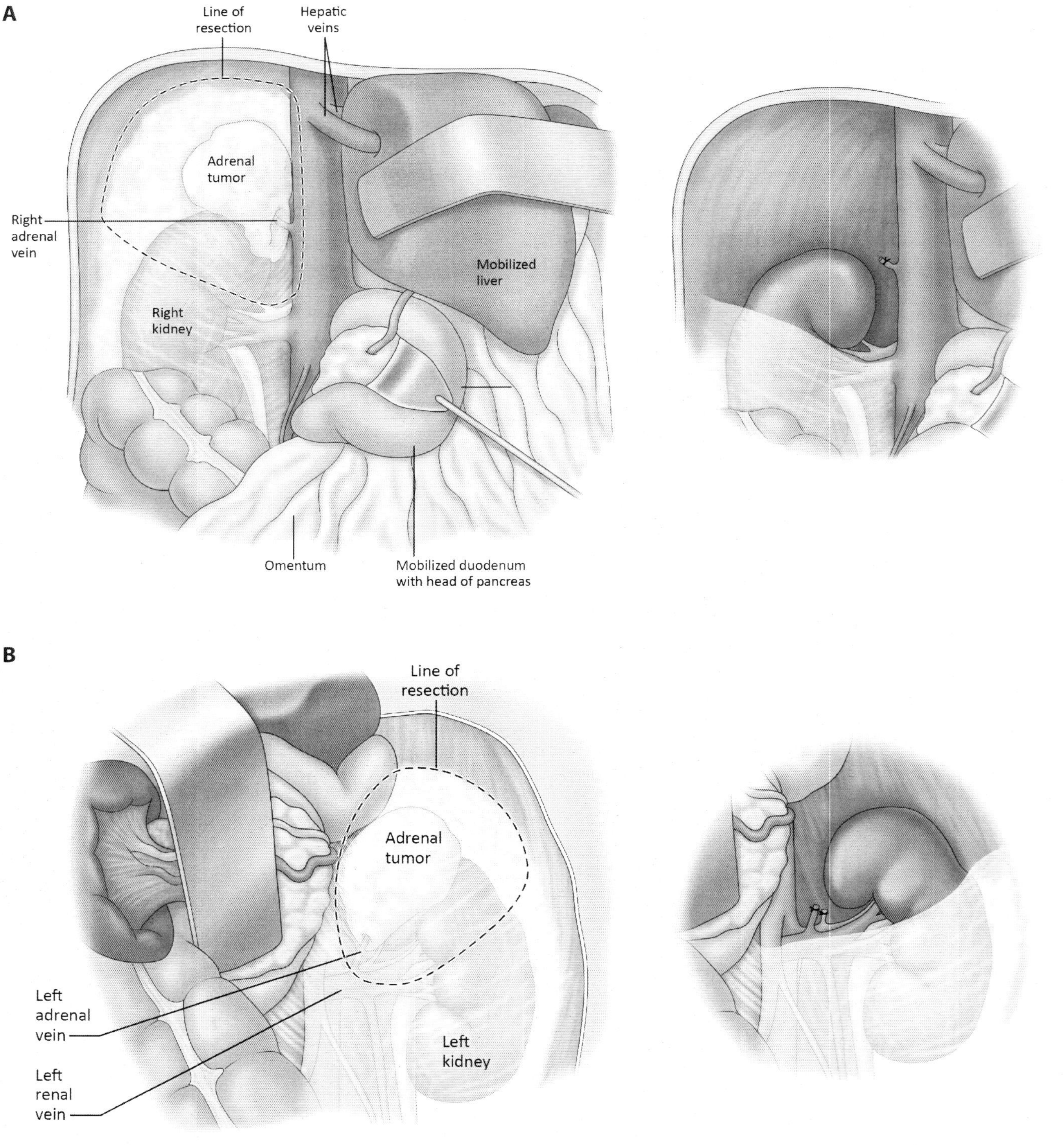

Figure 2 Margins of resection (as indicated by dashed line) including periadrenal adipose tissue for right (**A**) and left (**B**) adrenalectomy.

Note O: Adjacent Organs Resected if Suspected of Invasion

Explanatory Comments: Direct invasion of periadrenal organs is common, and the incidence of multiorgan resection at the time of adrenalectomy is as high as 40%. An artificial plane of resection between the primary tumor and adjacent organ should not be created when one no longer exists as shedding of tumor cells leads to local recurrence and peritoneal dissemination. Organs and structures resected *en bloc* with the primary tumor will depend on the laterality of the tumor. Select "yes" or "no" for suspected invasion of the listed organs. "Yes" also applies if preoperatively there is radiographic evidence of invasion. Choose the organ(s) involved and denote "yes" or "no" as appropriate if *en bloc* resection is performed. If an artificial plane is created between the primary tumor and adjacent organ, select "no" for *en bloc* resection if the adjacent organ is removed separately. For additional details, please refer to the *Operative Standards for Cancer Surgery,* Volume 3, pages 73-142, and the *AJCC Cancer Staging Manual,* Eighth Edition.

Note P: Lymph Nodes Removed

Explanatory Comments: Regional lymph node metastasis in patients with adrenal cancer is associated with worse survival. Lymph node dissection for adrenal cancer constitutes removal of lymph nodes in the regions surrounding the affected adrenal gland and areas most prone to have regional metastatic nodal disease. The primary nodal regions most frequently found to harbor regional metastatic disease are the paracaval and para-aortic cranial regions. While prophylactic regional nodal dissection is not recommended within the ACS OSCS for adrenal cancer, therapeutic regional nodal dissection of involved nodal basins is recommended when suspicion or confirmation of metastatic nodal disease is identified by preoperative imaging and/or intraoperatively. Any lymph nodes removed should be labeled and sent to pathology, indicated using the SOR, and included in any other operative report.
NCDB coding instructions for Scope of Regional Lymph Node Surgery [1292], used to identify the removal, biopsy, or aspiration of regional lymph node(s) at the time of surgery of the primary site or during a separate surgical event, are detailed in the *STORE 2023* manual. NCDB coding instructions for Scope of Regional Lymph Node Surgery at this Facility [672] are also detailed in the *STORE 2023* manual.

Note Q: Venous Thrombectomy

Explanatory Comments: Venous tumor thrombus may be identified preoperatively on cross-sectional imaging or identified intraoperatively. If venous thrombectomy is performed, select "yes." Select "no" if no venous thrombectomy is performed. For additional details, please refer to the *Operative Standards for Cancer Surgery,* Volume 3, pages 73-142, and the *AJCC Cancer Staging Manual,* Eighth Edition.

Note R: Venous Reconstruction

Explanatory Comments: Venous reconstruction may be necessary as a result of direct invasion by the primary tumor or other factors. The selection of the appropriate reconstruction technique depends on the degree of involvement of the vessel. Mobile tumor thrombus with no or minimal involvement of the wall of the vein may be simply extracted by venotomy and primary repair, while more extensive involvement may require reconstruction with either a patch (autologous, bovine pericardium, synthetic material) or interposition graft. In cases where the inferior vena cava (IVC) is unable to be reconstructed, segmental resection with ligation of the IVC may be performed. For additional details, please refer to the *Operative Standards for Cancer Surgery,* Volume 3, pages 73-142, and the *AJCC Cancer Staging Manual,* Eighth Edition.

Note S: Need for Vascular Bypass

Explanatory Comments: Vascular bypass to provide continued perfusion of vital structures and facilitate complete tumor resection in an oncologically appropriate manner may be required during resection of adrenal cancers. The need for vascular bypass is dictated both by patient factors, tolerance of clamping of the vasculature, and the location as it relates to the vena cava and hepatic veins. Thrombectomy or vena cava resection inferior to the hepatic veins most often can be managed without the need for vascular bypass. Venovenous bypass may be required for hemodynamically unstable patients and those requiring clamping of the IVC at the level of or a location superior to the hepatic veins. In those with tumor thrombus extending superiorly such that safe distal control of the IVC cannot be established (thrombus extending to and into the right atrium), cardiopulmonary bypass with or without hypothermic circulatory arrest or venovenous bypass may be required. For additional details, please refer to the *Operative Standards for Cancer Surgery,* Volume 3, pages 73-142, and the *AJCC Cancer Staging Manual,* Eighth Edition.

Note T: Resection of Metastatic Disease

Explanatory Comments: Multivisceral resection is a very common occurrence in operations done for adrenocortical carcinoma. This is less often required for malignancy pheochromocytomas. This is typically performed because of direct local invasion or vascular involvement of adjacent organs. In this section, please indicate any and all additional organs that are resected with the specimen. For kidney involvement, please indicate if a complete or partial nephrectomy was performed.

Note U: Capsular Disruption of Tumor

Explanatory Comments: Surgery for primary adrenal cancers requires delicate dissection and tissue handling of the tumor, its surrounding envelope of retroperitoneal adipose tissue, and Gerota's fascia. In this section, please note if the capsule of the tumor was disrupted during the operation. If capsular disruption occurred, please note if there was spillage of tumor fragments into the retroperitoneum or peritoneal cavity.

Note V: Clinical Resection Status

Explanatory Comments: The operative report must document any findings of gross residual disease at the end of the case. Definitions for R Designation from the AJCC are summarized below in Table 3.

Patients with microscopically or grossly positive margins (R1 or R2) have a statistically higher risk of recurrence and/or disease specific death. For additional details, please refer to the *Operative Standards for Cancer Surgery,* Volume 3, pages 73-142, and the *AJCC Cancer Staging Manual,* Eighth Edition.

Table 3. Definition of R Designation (Residual Tumor After Treatment)

R	R Definition
R0	No residual tumor
R1	Microscopic residual tumor
R2	Macroscopic residual tumor at the primary cancer site or regional nodal sites (This designation is not used to indicate metastatic disease identified but not resected at surgical exploration.)

AJCC Cancer Staging Manual, Eighth Edition, Chapter 1 (Principles of Cancer Staging)

Section 3: Additional Procedure Details

Note W: Additional Procedures

Explanatory Comments: The following fields have been included for the SOR to represent a complete record of information so that it not only will fulfill surgeon and institutional documentation needs, but also can fulfill regulatory requirements. The inclusion of open-text narrative fields provides sufficient flexibility for all aspects of surgical care to be recorded and for multiple functions, such as registry submission and generation of billing codes, to be permissible.

Note X: Additional Surgical Variables

Explanatory Comments: This section is provided to add additional surgical variables to the synoptic report that are not listed. Please describe the additional variables in the narrative box (if applicable).

Note Y: Intraoperative Complications

Explanatory Comments: Surgery for primary adrenal cancers can involve large incisions and complex multivisceral resection. It is important to review and document the nature of any intraoperative complications that arise, including those that result from specific technical maneuvers as well as those resulting from physiologic derangements, anesthesia-related complications, patient positioning, etc. In this section, document the specific nature of any intraoperative complication including but not limited to injury to adjacent organs (spleen, pancreas, colon, liver, kidney, etc.), blood vessels (IVC, renal vessels, splenic vessels, aorta), ureters, diaphragm, pneumothorax, etc. The surgeon should also indicate complications of a physiologic nature such as myocardial infarction, dysrhythmia, pulmonary embolus, coagulopathy, and/or transfusion of any blood products.

References

1. Amin MB, Edge SB, Greene FL, et al, eds. *AJCC Cancer Staging Manual*. 8th edit. New York, NY: Springer; 2017.
2. Commission on Cancer. *Standards for Oncology Registry Entry (STORE)*. Chicago, IL: American College of Surgeons; 2023.
3. Hunt KK, Katz MH, Veeramachaneni N, et al. *Operative Standards for Cancer Surgery*. Vol 3. Chicago, IL: Wolters Kluwer; 2023.

Made in United States
North Haven, CT
05 November 2026

21767750R00015